TTC

TO ...

BFP⁺

THE GUIDE TO LEARNING YOUR BODY'S SIGNALS WHEN TRYING TO CONCEIVE

⁺ TRYING TO CONCEIVE TO...BIG FAT POSITIVE ⁺

ISBN: 978-1975606534
ISBN-13: 1975606531

TABLE OF CONTENTS

PART I - INTRODUCTION

A. OVERVIEW

Are you TTC?

When was your LMP?

How long is your LP?

These are just a few of the many questions and acronyms you'll read about when trying to conceive (TTC). This guide will help put these into context while you learn your fertility signals and unravel some of the mystery surrounding TTC.

It can be overwhelming trying to digest all the advice from so many different TTC sources. I wrote this guide so you can have the most valuable information in one place for the best odds of getting a positive home pregnancy test (HPT+ = Big Fat Positive (BFP)). Even if you aren't planning to TTC right away, this guide will educate you and become an invaluable resource for when you are ready.

I've helped many women who, when starting on this journey, were disappointed when they didn't get their BFP right away after stopping birth control and having unprotected sex ("baby dance"=BD). The only things they really knew about their cycles were how long their periods ("Aunt Flow"=AF) lasted and when to expect the next one.

There are medical reasons for the changes during your monthly cycle, such as fluctuating hormones but this guide doesn't delve into those. This is a reference tool to help you learn and recognize your body's fertile signals, pinpoint ovulation, and the optimal time to BD, which will help you go from TTC to BFP+!

B. WHY I WROTE THIS GUIDE (A BIT ABOUT ME)

I'm the sole parent of three amazing kids who are growing up way too fast and are making me miss the TTC days! During the TTC-phase of my life, I got pregnant five times in five years, which I attribute to obsessively learning all about my fertility.

My first BFP came as a complete shock because my husband and I were using birth control at the time. I didn't know anything about my cycles or fertility, other than my period came every 35 days. After I had my son, I caught "baby fever" and wanted to TTC as soon as possible. I started researching TTC and fertility cues since I had never actively tried to get pregnant before. Turns out I had plenty of time to learn because my fertility took a while to return while I was breastfeeding (BF). I had a lot of 'false-starts' but got pregnant before my post-partum AF (PPAF) returned! I pinpointed my first postpartum ovulation (PPO) by learning all my body's fertility signs and tracking them daily from the time my son was a few months old. These signs had been there all along but I had never paid attention to them.

I went to my OB that day to confirm my pregnancy. Her test was negative and she told me the HPT was likely defective, and advised me to wait to until my PPAF arrived before TTC. I made her a deal that if I came back in a few days and got a BFP in her office, she would owe me lunch. Who says there's no free lunch?!

Even though my OB was excited for me, she never asked how I was so sure about being pregnant. Her only comment was "you must have had a lot of sex last month!" I didn't tell her that my husband had been traveling all month and we only BD one time.

I still can't believe I only started learning about cervical mucus (CM), cervical position (CP), luteal phase (LP), and basal body temperature (BBT) at the age of 31, and after having my first child! I couldn't help but think to myself, "This Really Works! Why didn't I know about this sooner?!"

I became so fascinated with cycles, fertility, and TTC that I became an on-line moderator for TTC message boards. I also became a consultant, working privately with posters, lurkers, their friends, as well as local friends and family. After countless women told me this was the first time they were learning about their fertility signs, I decided to write this guide to help even more women. This guide should help healthy women with normal cycles learn about their bodies and assist them in getting pregnant.

If after reading this guide, tracking your cycle, and TTC unsuccessfully for a few months, you should make an appointment with your OB.

I sincerely hope this helps you go from TTC to BFP!

C. PRE-TEEN GIRLS

Although this guide is for women TTC, I feel strongly that parts of this guide should be taught to pre-teen girls when they start menstruating. It's disheartening to me that girls aren't taught more about their bodies. I know it might seem weird to talk about pre-teen girls in a TTC book but I feel very strongly that girls need to start knowing their bodies, cycles, and symptoms when they get their first AF, but for very different reasons than TTC. Girls should be taught about the different discharge and feelings that occur during the month. Being aware will hopefully give girls confidence. So many are uncomfortable with, and shy about, their bodies. Wouldn't it be amazing if we taught girls that their menstruation cycle is normal and to embrace what their bodies are doing? When women complain about 'that time of the month', I tell them I'm happy when I get AF because it tells me my body is working properly. This hatred over periods gets passed down to their daughters. I believe if pre-teen girls are taught about different discharge, and to track their AF so they aren't unprepared when their periods arrive, they will feel more in-control of their bodies and maybe end the negative stigma.

I remember when I was in 9th grade during a final exam, I felt a rush of liquid gush out of me. I was worried it was my period but thought that I just had it two weeks before. I didn't want to stand up if I was having AF because I wasn't prepared for it. I waited until the entire class left, ran into the bathroom, and saw white, gooey discharge. I had no idea if that was normal, or if I had some weird infection. No one had talked to me about CM once I had regular periods. It wasn't until TTC that I realized that discharge was EWCM. Had I known about CM and EWCM at the time, I wouldn't have felt so confused and embarrassed.

Although my daughter hasn't reached puberty yet, I plan to go over aspects of this guide with her when she gets her period. I'm not going to discuss TTC, but I want her to become comfortable and aware of the body changes to that will come when she starts her period. Then, when she's *much* older, and decides to TTC, she will be ahead of the game!

D. LET'S GET STARTED...

As discussed, you probably didn't learn a lot during your pre-teen years about your monthly cycle aside from being told once you get your period your breasts will get larger and body hair will start sprouting. A few years later, people told you to start using birth control when you become sexually active because of the possibility of becoming pregnant.

Fast forward to when you're ready to TTC and don't know much more than to stop using birth control and BD as much as possible.

If you've been trying to avoid (TTA) getting pregnant the only thing you really had to remember was to use a birth control method. You knew the protection was working when you got your AF at the end of the month.

The first day of regular menstrual flow, meaning there is bleeding that needs a pad or tampon, is referred to as cycle day one (CD 1). Spotting is considered the last days of the previous cycle.

Although all women start counting their cycle days on CD 1, what happens during the cycle varies. An over-simplification of a woman's cycle is that it's 28 days with the following breakdown:

CD 1 – First day of Period (AF)

CD 14 – Ovulation

CD 28 – Last day of cycle before period starts the next day.

The 28-day cycle is a generalization and not necessarily typical. Sometimes the length of time between CD 1 to ovulation is longer or shorter than 14 days. There are some women who have gotten pregnant during their AF because they ovulated very early in their cycle.

The time between ovulation and AF is called the luteal phase (LP) and can be longer or shorter than 14 days (see Part II. C). The only way to know what's normal for you is to track your individual cycle.

Knowing when you ovulate is key to getting pregnant. It's possible to get pregnant by having sex 3-to-4 days before actual ovulation, as well as a day after ovulation. For example, if you ovulate on CD 14, you could BD only on CD 10 and still have a chance of pregnancy. This is because some sperm can survive in your body for 3-to-4 days. (side note: female sperm are said to live longer than male sperm so those trying for a specific gender try to time sex based on this). However, your odds of getting pregnant typically increase by BD within 1-to-2 days before ovulation because once the egg is released from your ovaries it needs to be fertilized within 24 hours. In addition, newer (more recent) sperm is heartier.

PART II – SPECIFIC BODY CUES

A. CM

Cervical mucus (CM) is vaginal discharge that varies throughout the month. Some common CM observations are dry, sticky, snot-like, yellow-tinged, creamy, or clear. Once your menstrual bleeding ends pay close attention to your CM because it's a significant factor in figuring out when your body is gearing up to ovulate.

Right after AF ends, CM will be scant, dry, sticky, and/or flaky, or could be white and a bit chalky. A few days later, CM becomes moist, snot-like and gooey, and will break apart if you try to stretch it. About a day or two before ovulation, your CM will become wet, clear (but might have a white-tinge), elastic, and stretchy. EWCM looks and feels like raw egg whites, and is designed help carry sperm to the egg, and protect the sperm by keeping it alive until the egg is released.

To differentiate fertile EWCM from other CM, residual semen, or lubricant after BD, collect a sample between your finger tips and thumb and separate your fingers; EWCM will stretch a few inches without breaking, while clear CM and semen will break apart almost immediately. Another way to tell the difference between semen and EWCM is to use the water test. Collect a sample and put it in water; if it floats or dissolves, it's semen; if it forms a ball and/or sinks, it's EWCM.

If you don't have noticeable CM, especially EWCM, make sure you're well-hydrated. Drink lot of fluids, including water, grapefruit, or pineapple juice, or decaffeinated green tea, all which have been proven to increase CM. Other remedies are to cut down or eliminate caffeine, take a teaspoon of cough syrup 2x daily between the time menstruation ends and ovulation, take Evening Primrose Oil (EPO) starting with low-doses of 500mg, 3x daily (but make sure to stop taking EPO once you've ovulated), avoid antihistamines, and eat lots of vegetables, especially carrots.

If you're dry when BD, use a lubricant specially formulated for TTC. These targeted lubricants mimic EWCM that keep sperm alive and mobile, as opposed to commercial lubricant which can slow down, or kill off, sperm. Since these specialty lubricants can be expensive, save it for when you're nearing ovulation.

Just before AF is due, CM could dry up, turn white, or, sometimes as a sign of pregnancy, turn white with a yellow tinge. Keep tracking your CM until you get your AF or BFP!

B. LH SURGE / OPKS

OPKs measure the Luteinizing Hormone (LH) in your system and are positive when LH surges to its highest level during the month, about 12 hours before ovulation. OPKs can consistently show a second a second line, indicating there's LH in your system. Unlike HPTs which are considered positive whenever there is a second line on the test, an OPK is only positive when the test line is as dark as, or darker, than the control line. When the second line is equal to or darker than the control line, your LH surge is at its monthly peak, and ovulation is imminent. You can track other symptoms along with OPKs to confirm pending ovulation, such as the presence of EWCM.

When your OPK turns positive, you will likely ovulate within the next 12-to-24 hours. You should BD within that timeframe for the greatest chance of a BFP. An OPK quickly turns from negative to positive and back to negative, sometimes within a few hours, so start OPK testing when your CM transitions from dry to moist. Once your CM becomes EWCM, you should use the OPKs 2-to-3 times a day until it turns positive. Remember that it's still possible to get pregnant before you ovulate because sperm can live 3-to-4 days before ovulation, so don't obsess if you can't BD when you get the positive OPK, especially if you've BD in the days leading up to it. There's also a chance of pregnancy when you BD a day after ovulation, but it's still best to BD at least once between when you get a positive OPK and when the OPK turns negative.

You can stop using OPKs as soon as you get a positive OPK. Ovulation will be confirmed by EWCM drying up, and your BBT temperature will rise (see Part D BBT). If possible, continue BD until you have clear confirmation of ovulation.

If you or your spouse travel a lot, TTC can be even more frustrating, especially when you get a positive OPK and you can't be together. If you can start seeing a pattern of when you ovulate, try to plan on BD that time next month.

Once you get your BFP you might be wondering if this baby is a girl or a boy. At your 20-week ultrasound you can find out the gender and be on the pink team (pregnant with a girl), blue team (pregnant with a boy), or you can choose not to find out and be a member of the green team. Sometimes you can make an educated guess by looking back at your chart. If you BD a few days before ovulation occurred, you might be having a girl since female sperm swim slower but live longer. If you only BD at ovulation, odds are more in favor of a boy because the male sperm swim very fast but die quickly, so if the egg was going to be released a few hours after BD, there's a good chance it was the male sperm up there waiting to meet the egg! Of course, this isn't an exact science, but it's fun to guess and when you find out for certain, check back with your chart to see if you were right!

C. LP AND THE 2WW

The LP is also known as the 2 Week Wait (2WW), because once you've ovulated you need to wait about two weeks before you can confidently test for pregnancy or find out you're not pregnant when AF arrives. If you're pregnant, the pregnancy hormone human chorionic gonadotropin (HCG) needs to build up in your system before it will register on a HPT. HCG doubles every 48 hours and most HPTs are will register HCG at 20 or above, which translates to roughly 12 DPO.

It's not important to your fertility what CD you ovulate. You could have a short monthly cycle and ovulate early with a long LP, or a long cycle and ovulate sooner, or later, in your cycle and have a long LP. For instance, my cycles are 35 days and I typically ovulate on CD 21, so I ovulate 'late' according to the 28 Day Cycle but have a typical 14-day LP. LP is *very* important to your fertility. Your LP should be at least 9-10 days long. A short LP doesn't give your uterine lining time to thicken and create an ideal environment for pregnancy, and doesn't give the egg enough time to implant. (see Part C for LP)

The 2WW isn't exactly 14 days and you can start testing with a HPT as soon as 8 DPO. Most women try to wait until 10 DPO to test so they don't have to deal with a false (or actual) BFN.

During your 2WW continue to track your BBT, monitor CP and CM, and note any other symptoms.

If you're an early tester, don't be discouraged by a BFN, especially before 12 DPO. Implantation might occur later during LP, meaning that HCG starts building in your system later than if it occurred during ovulation and will take longer to register on a HPT.

If you don't have HPTs but have extra OPKs, and you really want to start peeing on a stick (POAS) sooner than 10 DPO, you can use an OPK. Sometimes when you're pregnant, an OPK will turn positive late in your cycle (although the reverse is not true: a HPT can't be substituted for an OPK). If you have already ovulated and are expecting your AF, getting a positive OPK could indicate that you're pregnant!

About 7 DPO you could have a day of spotting which could indicate a short LP, or it could be due to implantation! If you spot for a day and then CM goes back to white, clear, or dry, the spotting could have been from implantation. Other clues this could be implantation spotting are: implantation pattern (See Part D: BBT), CM tinged pink, one episode of spotting, brownish CM along with nausea, breast / nipple sensitivity, fatigue, and increased urination. If you have the mucous-y CM when you're nearing AF, it could be the mucous plug forming – another pregnancy sign. Sometimes CM is white with a yellow tinge for the same reason. If your LP is short and you get your AF before 10 DPO, you can try using some of the supplements listed in Part V. Otherwise, talk to your OB about prescription solutions.

D. BBT

Taking your basal body temperature (BBT) lets you know if you are pre- or post-ovulation within your cycle, but it doesn't tell you when you're about to ovulate. Tracking your BBT is more about confirming ovulation than telling you when to BD. Your BBT is unique to you, meaning somebody else's resting BBT could be higher or lower than yours. It's important to know your pre-ovulation temperature so that you will be able to determine when you ovulated. When TTC, BBT needs to be taken right when you wake up, before getting out of bed, around the same time every morning, and after being at rest for at least a few hours.

Post-ovulation temperature can be different for everyone but it's typically about 1to-1 $^{1/4}*$ higher than pre-ovulation. If, during the last few days of your cycle, your BBT drops back to pre-ovulation levels, AF should arrive soon. If your BBT stays at post-ovulation levels after AF was due, you could be pregnant and your BBT will remain elevated throughout your pregnancy.

The plotting of all the BBT can form few different patterns. One pattern is that your post-ovulation BBT stays relatively constant. This is a typical biphasic chart with two ranges of BBT: lower pre-ovulation and higher post-ovulation temperatures. Another pattern is a triphasic chart which has three different ranges: lower pre-ovulation, higher post-ovulation and then another temperature rise above the previous post-ovulation BBT. Lastly, a BBT drop below, or near pre-ovulation, levels for a day, especially accompanied by light spotting, and then rises back up the next day, could be an implantation pattern. You might assume that because your BBT dropped and you're spotting that your AF is arriving early, but don't get discouraged - you might soon get a BFP!

A biphasic, triphasic, or an implantation dip pattern doesn't guarantee pregnancy but are signs you've ovulated. Continue to note your BBT regardless, and if it remains high for 7-10 days post-ovulation, take go POAS!

If you do get a BFP, you'll have a more precise estimated due date (EDD) than the doctor, who calculates your EDD from the beginning of your last menstrual period (LMP). The difference between their EDD and your EDD is that yours is based on your ovulation date and theirs starts from CD 1 and assumes the 28-day cycle with ovulation on CD 14. The EDD you calculate could also be a few days off because implantation could have taken place a few days or even a week after you ovulated. That's why it's called an estimation even when you know your ovulation date.

Your body gearing up for AF or BFP could have very similar signs – bloating, spotting, tender breasts, breakouts, white/yellow CM – but one main difference is that your post-ovulation BBT remains elevated after AF is due. You can start testing if your BBT remains high about 7 DPO but don't be discouraged by an early BFN. Typically, a HPT will be accurate around 12-14 DPO.

Note: You don't need a special BBT thermometer. Any thermometer will work well if you take your temperature at the same time every day.

E. CP

Your CP is another physical change that takes place during the month. CP is lowest at the beginning of your cycle (during AF) then slowly rises, peaking during ovulation. CP will lower again at the end of your cycle if you aren't pregnant or stay elevated if you are. If

BD has ever been painful or uncomfortable for you, especially at the beginning or end of the month, it could be due to low CP.

You can check your CP by inserting your fingers into your vagina, but make sure they are clean so you don't introduce bacteria and risk infection. A good practice is to check CP in the shower or bath.

Closer to ovulation, your CP will begin to rise and you will have to reach farther to find it. When your body is gearing up to ovulate, your CP is at its highest (and softest) for the month and you might not be able to reach it. At this point you should notice that your CM has become EWCM. This is an ideal time to BD.

After ovulation, your CP will lower back down, sometimes within a few hours. Near the end of your cycle, if you're not pregnant, your CP will once again be very low (and hard). However, if you're pregnant your CP will remain high.

F. SENSATIONS

Some women can feel symptoms of ovulation when the egg is being released. Once you learn your cycle and really start paying attention to the signs, you might realize that you've been feeling these sensations but blamed them on other things, such as gas, cramps, or stomach aches. Once you hone in on the timing of ovulation, you might be able to feel the many twinges, pinches, aches, heaviness and fullness, and / or cramps pinches during ovulation!

If you have both ovaries, ovulation can take place on either side each month. There is no pattern to which ovary will release an egg. Ovaries don't take turns each month. You can ovulate on the left OR right (or both) side each month so if you happen to feel sensations on one side the previous month, it doesn't mean you'll ovulate from the opposite side the next month. If you only have one ovary, you will ovulate every month from that side.

PART III – ADDITIONAL TOOLS

A. HPTS

HPTs detect if there is HCG in your system and are a great way to find out if you're pregnant without having to go to the doctor for a test. They can be expensive but ones sold on the internet (internet cheapies) or dollar stores are very accurate. HPTs give the best results with first morning urine (FMU) because it's usually the most concentrated.

B. CHARTING

So how do you keep track of all these symptoms throughout the month? Charting! (see sample in Part IX). Charting is an easy way to gather and notate all your daily. Charting also allows you to put in notes, which is important if you've been sick, had sleepless nights, woke up earlier than normal, or traveled to a different time zone. For instance, you might have the flu a week after AF ends and BBT will show high post-ovulation temperatures even though you haven't ovulated. If you've notated it on your chart you'll be able to see why there were higher temperatures so early in your cycle. Notes are extremely helpful when you can't remember why there is something that doesn't fit your typical pattern from a few weeks, a few months, ago.

There are numerous free online charting sites, as well as paper charts. By charting, you can see your monthly symptoms and activities at-a-glance and notice your unique patterns. Continue inputting your data every day and soon it will become second nature. As soon as you wake up, take your BBT and input it, if you BD make sure you add it into your chart, and throughout the day, notate your CM and CP, and any other symptoms as well.

PART IV – TTC WHILE BF

TTC while breastfeeding (BF) can be tricky. For many women (but not all), BF suppresses ovulation, which is why some are unable to get pregnant while BF. There are a few women who get PPAF shortly after giving birth but their cycles might not be regular and/or their LP is very short. Other women find that cycles take longer to return and normalize. If you're vigilant about observing your body's signals, it's possible to get pregnant from your first PPO and never get PPAF. However, charting while BF can be frustrating because your body can be prone to "fake-outs", where signs of fertility return but ovulation doesn't happen for weeks, months, or years depending how long you're BF and when your fertility returns. Sometimes you can speed up your fertility's return by changing the times you BF or cutting out a feeding (for older babies). You need be patient and trust that your fertility will return when your body is ready to carry another baby. For me, I used OPKs while BF my son because I wanted to catch my PPO and get pregnant before I got my PPAF. There were months where I had almost positive OPKs but didn't get a true positive OPK until my son was nearly 10 months old!

PART V – SUPPLEMENTS

The following are some common vitamins and supplements thought to help with TTC, though not all are scientifically proven. Some are off-label uses in mega doses (more than RDA), and some are homeopathic that are not FDA regulated. Always use caution when starting any supplement and talk to your OB. It's always best to get nutrients from real food when possible.

A. Anti-Oxidants can increase LP.
B. B vitamins may assist your ovaries in releasing an egg around ovulation:
   1. **B3** may prevent some miscarriages and birth defects. 18 mg max daily.
   2. **B6** may increase levels of progesterone which can help lengthen LP, necessary to maintain your pregnancy. (can also be found in green, leafy vegetables).
   3. **Folic Acid**, a B complex vitamin that is helpful to take before you even begin TTC, helps prevent some birth defects of the baby's brain and spinal cord.

4. **B12** may prevent severe birth defects (including neural tube defects), may prevent infertility, miscarriages, and preterm birth.

C. **Bromelain** is only found in pineapple and is thought to assist in implantation when eaten just before and during ovulation.

D. **Evening Primrose Oil (EPO)** helps increase CM, specifically EWCM.

E. **Omega-3 fatty acids** help ovaries release eggs, increase blood flow to the uterus, and balance out your hormones and help lengthen LP. They may assist with fetal brain development.

F. **Prenatal Vitamins** contain more folic acid and iron than regular daily vitamins.

1. **Folic acid** helps prevent neural tube defects.

2. **Iron** supports the baby's growth, development, and prevents anemia.

G. **Red Raspberry Leaf Tea** is a homeopathic supplement that contains a mix of B complex, calcium, iron, magnesium, and other vitamins thought to regulate irregular menstrual cycles and lengthen LP. When taken during pregnancy, helps with morning sickness, and promotes better circulation. Taking raspberry leaf is believed to help strengthen uterine muscles and tone the pelvic floor in preparation for childbirth, and even increases breastmilk supply.

H. **Vitamin C** can help make LP longer.

I. Vitamin E is found in the fluid around your developing eggs where deficiencies could cause fertility issues.

J. Vitex is a homeopathic herbal supplement that supports many gynecological imbalances, including lengthening LP.

PART VI – END OF CYCLE NON-PREGNANT VS. POSSIBLY PREGNANT

A. Not Pregnant:

1. CM dries up, is non-existent or spotting occurs a few days before AF
2. BBT drops to pre-ovulation temperature just before AF is due
3. CP goes back to being low and hard

B. Possibly Pregnant:

1. CM is white with yellow tinge, possibly 'snotty' in texture
2. BBT stays elevated at post-ovulation after AF is due
3. Implantation dip with a day of spotting
4. Triphasic chart
5. CP remains high and soft
6. Positive OPK towards end of cycle
7. Nausea, tender breasts and nipples, fatigue, increased urination

PART VII - ADDITIONAL SERVICES: CONSULTING AND MORE!

*If you feel you need more personalized instructions and analyses, I am available for private consultations. I would love the opportunity to work with you! My services include: reading, analyzing, and interpreting your chart one-time, weekly, or month-long, coaching, making suggestions, answering questions in a timely manner, tutoring, talking through frustrations, stress, and lending emotional support. I also have a private Facebook group for those who bought this guide and want to have a safe place to talk, ask questions, post charts and other images, and receive support from me and other women TTC. TTC can be fun and exciting, but it can also be stressful and, ironically, lonely and I want to help ease the stress and loneliness. If you feel stuck and want a personal, one-on-one consultation, please email me at: **TTCtoBFP@gmail.com**. Together, we can find the best course of action that serves your personal needs. I am honored that you have chosen my guide and can't wait to go on this journey with you. Even if you don't want to hire me, I would love to hear from you when you get your BFP!*

(Side note: I also sell inexpensive but accurate OPKs and HPT strips to my clients. Email me at: ttctobfp@gmail.com for more information. Remember, though, OPKs are not necessary if you're in tune with your CM, CP, body twinges and BBT).

PART VIII – GLOSSARY

AF - Aunt Flow = Period

BBT – Basal Body Temperature = your lowest body temperature in a 24-hour period.

BD – Baby Dance = Sex

BF - Breastfeeding

BFN – Big Fat Negative = negative pregnancy test

BFP – Big Fat Positive = positive pregnancy test

Blue Team – Pregnant with a Boy

Catching the first egg – Pregnant from the first ovulation after having a baby, before PPAF

CD - Cycle Day

Chart – a place to keep track of all activity during your cycle (see example below)

CM – Cervical Mucus

CP – Cervical Position

Day 1 – First Day of Regular Menstrual Bleeding

DPO – Days Past Ovulation

EDD – Estimated Due Date

EPO – Evening Primrose Oil

EWCM – Egg White Cervical Mucus = the most fertile CM

FMU – First Morning Urine

Green Team – Not Finding out the Gender of the Baby

HCG - Human Chorionic Gonadotropin Hormone = Pregnancy Hormone

HPT – Home Pregnancy Test

Internet Cheapies – cheap OPK and HPT strips bought online

IRL – In Real Life

LH - Luteinizing Hormone

LMP – Last Menstrual Period

LP – Luteal Phase = from ovulation to end of cycle or pregnancy

O – Ovulation

OPKs – Ovulation Predictor Kits = LH surge strips

Pink Team – Pregnant with a Girl

POAS – Pee on a Stick

PPAF - Postpartum Aunt Flow = first period after giving birth

PPO – Postpartum Ovulation

Triphasic Chart – three BBT levels: pre- and post-ovulation and 3rd temperature rise

TTA – Trying to Avoid

TTC – Trying to Conceive

2WW – 2 Week Wait = After ovulation, waiting for AF or BFP

PART IX - CHART SAMPLE

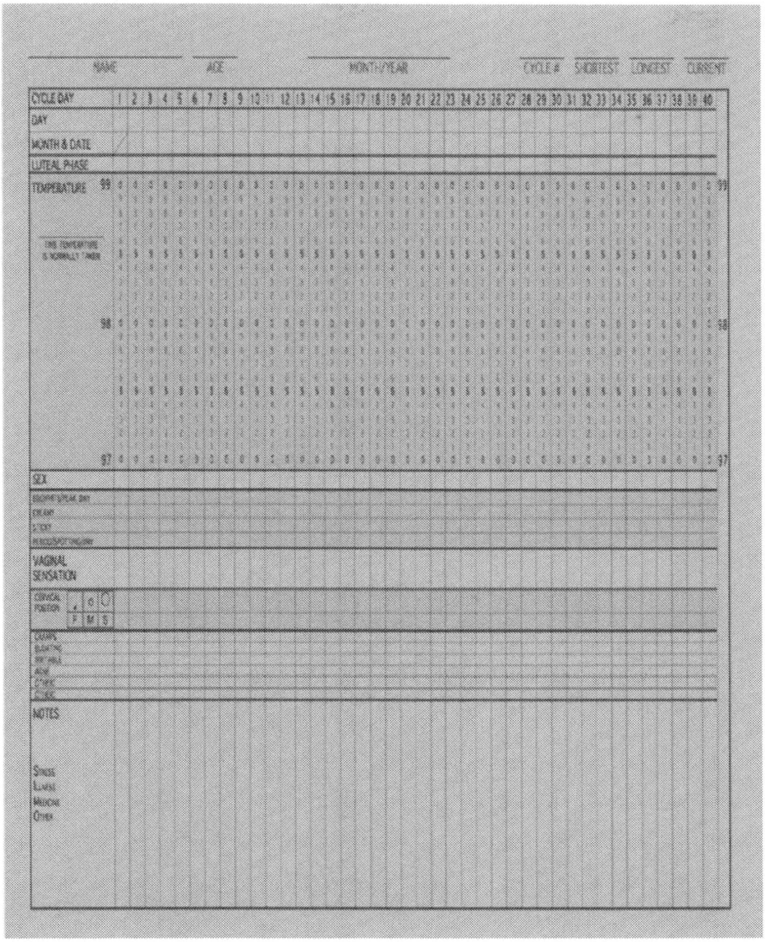

•

Made in the USA
Monee, IL
23 December 2020